Survival Guide:

15 Survival Strategies and Tips to Survive a Disaster

Disclamer: All photos used in this book, including the cover photo were made available under a <u>Attribution-NonCommercial-ShareAlike 2.0 Generic</u> and sourced from <u>Flickr</u>

Table of content

Introduction

Have you always wondered what you would do if a disaster has struck down and you have to survive without any help for a long period of time? In this book, you would be reading about surviving the toughest situations and training your mind on how to face fear and use it for your own advantage. You would learn what things you would need to survive in harsh circumstances. I have shared some ideas on storing enough water for your survival until help comes to you. I have discussed the preservation of food in one chapter too. There is a whole chapter about first aid in which I have tried my best to explain how to handle certain injuries and wounds when you have no help.

You cannot survival adverse situations if your mind if fearful. I have explained how you can face your fears and train your mind to be able to survive the scariest of situations. You would also read about basic survival skills needed to survive.

I have explained every strategy and tip in a way that it is easy for everyone to understand. You would also learn to defend yourself against people who, in order to survive, would try to harm you just to get to your supplies.

Disasters and bad times are a part of your lives and you will find this book really helpful in coping with such circumstances.

Chapter 1 - Must Have Survival Skills

There is just so much to learn when it comes to surviving in difficult circumstances. You would not even know where to start learning? I am going to share with you the basic survival skills that everybody should have if he/she wants to survive when the times are hard.

In this chapter, you would learn the 6 basic survival strategies that you need when the times are hard and adverse. Let's have a look at the 6 strategies.

Strategy# 1 - Your Attitude:

The number one strategy is your attitude. Your survival depends mostly on your attitude, how you handle different survival situations. Your attitude would decide if you would live or die. So you have to concentrate on your attitude first.

Let me share with you "The Rule of Threes". The rule is as follows,

- You can survive for 3 minutes without air

- You can only survive 3 hours without a regulated body temperature (a proper shelter)

- You can only live for 3 days without water

- You cannot live for more than 3 weeks without food

This rule also guides you about the important of different things for your survival.

Air>Shelter>Water>Food

Surviving a disaster also requires that you do not panic in the face of survival challenges. When you encounter a survival threat, remember this word, **SPEAR.**

Stop

Plan

Execute

Assess

Re-evaluate

To address a difficult and harsh situation, it is very important that you do everything in a calm manner and systematically. This will keep your body and mind fully focused on the matter at hand and keeps you from panicking or getting all sorts of negative vibes. With a resilient and strong attitude, your chances to survive any threat are greatly enhanced.

Strategy# 2 - Shelter:

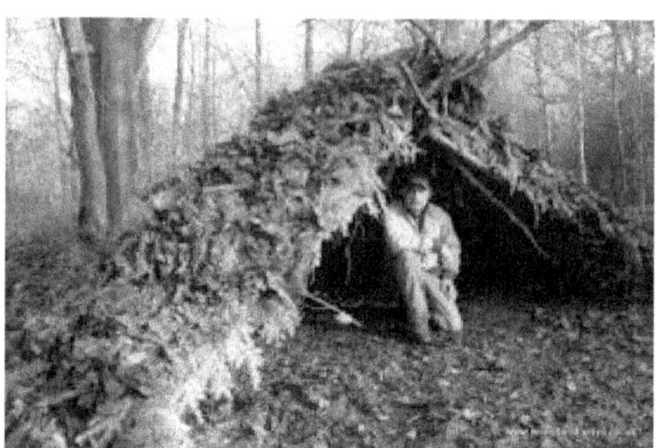

https://encrypted-tbn2.gstatic.com/images?
q=tbn:ANd9GcRF8qB9H3vuuHEnjADysDjyIoAjIujk-otufWJ-
TyzkF6aoespz

Shelter is very important when you face a survival situation. How? When you are in a survival situation and you don't have a proper shelter, you would be exposed to different elements that may harm your body and make you weak physically and mentally. So you should be able to build a shelter for you to survive any potential harsh condition. It is paramount that you avoid heat loss in your body and in hot circumstances; you have to keep yourself hydrated and prevent water loss in your body to keep you going on. You can build a shelter considering the following points,

- The location should be away from any hazards and near materials that you would need.

- The shelter should be able to insulate you from ground, rain, wind, sun etc.

- The shelter should be near a heat source.

There are many types of natural shelters you can consider when facing a survival threat. You can take shelter in a cave or a hollow stump. Building a shelter with logs is also useful. In cold areas, building a snow hut is very useful. A debris hut is the most practical shelter that you can build to live in the face of potential survival threats.

Strategy# 3 - Water:

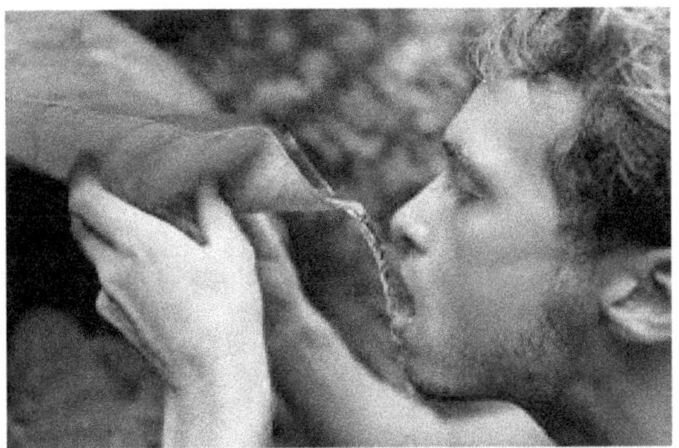

https://encrypted-tbn0.gstatic.com/images?q=tbn:ANd9GcQ98W8WmmEtZ7SXDXEg6XoIX-kPmkpHlF6BKJKRUKyqCxTV6Hb2qw

A human body consists mainly of water, up to 78%. This is why water is more important than food or fire. In ideal situations, a person consumes at least a gallon of water daily. People who survive the destruction caused by the disasters, often die because of dehydration or drinking unclean and unhealthy water. Unclean water can have various fatal bacteria, germs and pathogens. In addition to germs and pathogens, many streams and lakes contain industrial and agricultural waste which is also a cause of death because such water contains metals or elements that are seriously harmful for a human body. The best sources of water that are pure and harmless to human body are springs and small water tributaries. You can also collect morning dew which is pure too.

Filtering pumps and chemical treatments like iodine are the most popular ways of cleaning water before drinking it. If you have access to these elements, you would not have to worry about the water problem. There are many natural herbs that can clean water from germs and bacteria. Grapefruit seed extract is a very famous herbal water purifier but, there is still research going on, if it is 100% useful or not. The best way to purify water is to boil it. Cook water until big bubbles start to come to the top. Then keep boiling the water for 2-3 minutes will ensure that all the germs and bacteria are dead.

You can survive for weeks if you have an upright attitude, a good shelter and if you are drinking clean water.

Strategy# 4 - Fire:

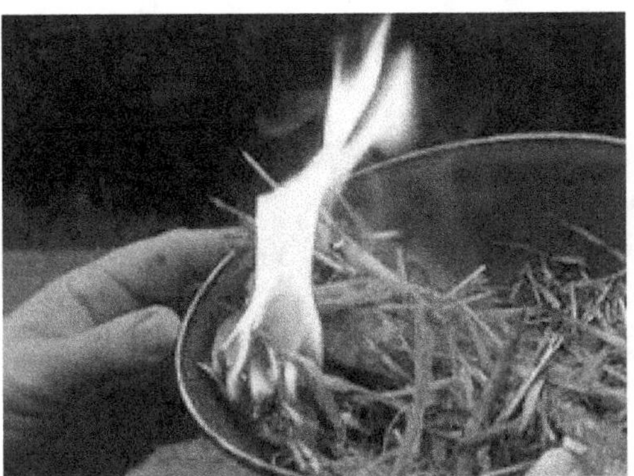

https://encrypted-tbn3.gstatic.com/images?
q=tbn:ANd9GcRG9quoeYd8RegoaUBTI5faOHx8sZSVCeEe_1v_XxV33FV
8EUHDZw

Fire is very important when you are facing a survival situation. It helps keep your body and shelter warm. You can dry your clothes, boil water and cook food for yourself with fires. Fire is also important to give you a sense of security and safety in a survival situation because different wild animals and preys can be scared off by fire.

It is ideal to carry fir starting tools with you almost all the time because who knows when you would be facing a survival condition. Keep a lighter with you, or matches, flint or steel etc. In adverse weather, it would be challenging to start a fire even if you have any of these implements. It is very important that you learn some basic fire-making skills to keep yourself ready if a disaster strikes down and you have to survive difficult times. Starting fire by friction is the most popular way of starting a fire. The most famous fire-making methods are bow drill method, fire plough method and fire saw method etc.

Strategy# 5 - Food:

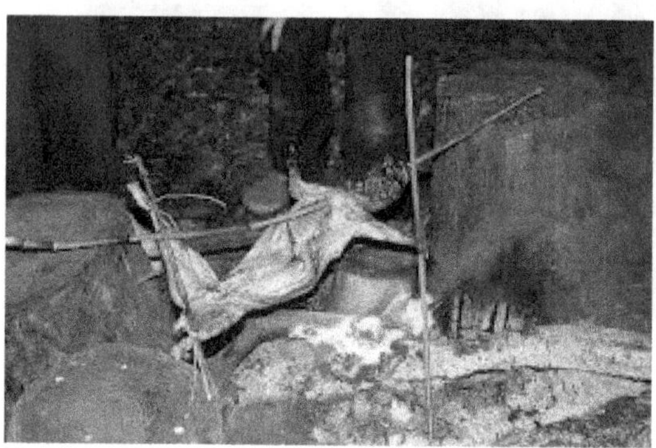

https://encrypted-tbn2.gstatic.com/images?
q=tbn:ANd9GcRwQZj3dICEGanxRNHuyqvFfuC8vPCK6WeJkK_qSsYJ3
WyN9zLZ

This strategy is about being able to identify different plants that you can eat. As compared to water and shelter, you can survive longer without food. You can survive without food for 3 weeks. But you would become weak still. Our environment is full of different eatables if you just know what to eat. Wild plants are a great source of nutritional food but you have to be very careful because there are fruits and berries and herb that are poisonous too. So make sure you know what you are going to what when you are facing a survival challenge.

I have a list of plants that can be a god source of nutritional food for you,

- Cattail – You can eat the roots, shoots and the pollen heads.

- Conifers – You can eat the inner bark which is called the Cambium. It is full of sugars, starches and calories. You can find this on most of the evergreen and cone-bearing trees. Yew is poisonous.

- Grasses – You can drink the juices from the leaves. They are very nutritious. The root corm, you can roast and eat.

- Oaks –Leach the tannic acids from acorns and eat them. Acorns are a good source of fats, proteins and calories for you.

PRECAUTION: Use field guides to identify different roots, herbs and plants because there are many plants that are eatable but they have poisonous identical too that are exactly the same. So if you are not sure about a plant, don't eat it.

Strategy# 6 - Naturalistic Knowledge:

The sixth skill that you need to survive a natural disaster is to have naturalistic knowledge. The more you know about nature, the more chances are of your survival. If you have wildlife tracking skills, it would be easy for you to catch game for your food and hunt. If you know different herbs and plants, it would be easy for you to find the right food to eat and use different herbs to treat different illnesses and injuries. Having a good knowledge about your body and how different organs are inter-related can help a lot in a survival situation. You would be able to utilize your resources in a more useful manner.

You should have a basic knowledge about natural sciences too like Botany, Geology, Zoology, Ecology etc.

The 6 strategies that I have discussed in this chapter are the most important things for your survival. If you can take care of these 6 points, you would be able to survive longer than anybody else.

Chapter 2 - Learn First Aid to Handle Injuries

In this chapter, I have given the next 2 important tips and strategies need for survival.

Strategy# 7 - Knowing different injuries and wounds and how to take care of them

Strategy# 8 - Medications to keep with you to treat different injuries

In a survival situation, you will not have access to hospitals or medicines. Your best hope would be your own self. Which means you should be able to provide first aid to yourself and to others if need be. I have explained here about different basic injuries and wounds and how you can recognize them and treat them.

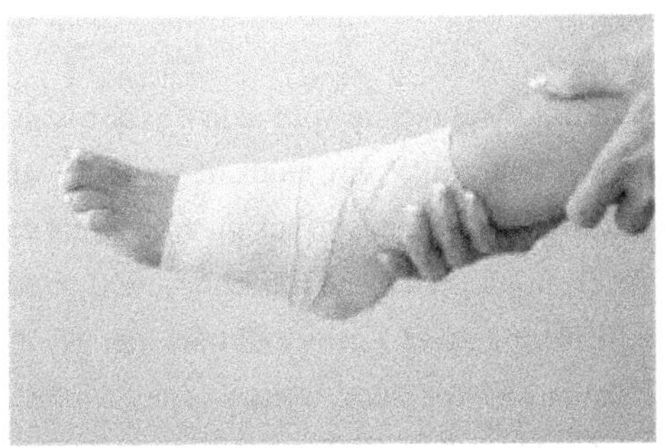

https://encrypted-tbn3.gstatic.com/images?
q=tbn:ANd9GcQYwVqrSrAUnO8kYpLKXhGWkbASGg9k9X31hTE
yXsk7zPo6GPFdDQ

What is an injury?

Any damage to your body is an injury. These are caused by accidents, hits, falls, bites, cuts, weapons etc. Injuries can be minor as well as fatal.

Here is a list of different kinds of injuries and how you can take care of them,

- Wounds

- Bruises

- Burns

- Dislocations

- Sprains and strains

Wounds - When an injury opens up your skin or your body tissues, it's called a wound. Cuts, scrapes etc are different kinds of wounds. Minor wounds are not serious but you have to clean them so that they don't get infected. You can use clean water to first clean all the blood from the wound and then you can use an antiseptic to keep it from getting germs and bacteria. Then you can cover it up with a clean bandage or piece of cloth. Deeper wounds need to be stitched. To be able to do that you should get first-aid lessons.

Bruises - It is also called a contusion or Ecchymoses. A bruise is an injury that happens when your blood is trapped under your skin. It happens when the impact cruses the blood vessel but the skin doesn't open up to get the blood out. So the blood gets trapped under your skin when it doesn't find a way to get out.

Such injuries are painful and the effected part might get swollen. You can get bruises on your skin, you muscles or even your bones. Bone bruises are the most serious ones.

How to treat bruises?

Bruises are reddish in colour and they turn purple or greenish before they heal. Bruises take months to heal but you can reduce the effect by applying ice on the affected area and lifting the part above your heart.

Burns – Burns are caused by the exposure of heat, chemicals or radiations to your body. Burns damage your skin and body tissues. Internal burns are also caused when you inhale in smoke or flammable gasses.

Burns are of three types,

- First-degree burns are when only the outer skin is damaged.

- Second-degree burns are when the next layer of your outer skin is damaged too.

- Third-degree burns are when the damage is too deep and the tissues are burnt too.

How to treat burns?

In case of minor burns, make sure the burned are doesn't get infected. Clean the injury and apply antibiotic creams on the area. Burns are very much prone to getting infected because the protective barrier of your skin is broken. So make sure the wound is clean and covered. Apply calamine lotion on the burnt area.

Dislocations - It is when the ends of your bones are dislocated. This happens as a result of a fall or a blow. When your bones are dislocated, it is visible and the area is usually swollen. You won't be able to move the dislocated part.

The best way to locate the bone back to the normal position is to do just push it back to the right place. This requires learning how to do it. After the dislocated joint has been returned to normal position, use a splint or a sling to keep it there and let the bones heal for a few days or weeks.

Sprains and Strains – These can happen as a result of falling, twisting or getting hit. A sprain happened when ligaments are stretched or torn. Ligaments are the tissues that are a connection between bones and the joint. The part will swell up and get bruised.

When a muscle or tendon is torn or stretched, it's called strain. Tendons are tissues that tear if you twist or pull your body part too hard, the muscles would swell and cause pain and you would get muscles spasms too as a result of a strain.

How to treat sprains and strains?

To treat sprains and strains, you should ice the area and wear a bandage or something that would compress the area. Later when the effects of the sprain or strain are fading, you can start doing minor exercises.

What do you need to treat different injuries?

https://encrypted-tbn2.gstatic.com/images?q=tbn:ANd9GcQRlQdECjVQXGTjI1XzKWXP-Zh_ib7dEueMYVVzdcrxRsgzaFKx

You should also know what you would need to treat different sorts of injuries with. This is a proven effective tip as you would be keeping medication that would help you survive different injuries and wounds. You should keep the following medications with you,

- Antibiotic ointment - To prevent minor wounds or injuries from getting infected

- Hydrocortisone cream - To reduce chemical reactions on the skin

- Calamine lotion - To relieve pain and prevent itching caused by poison, insect bites, burns or rashes

- Antihistamine, such as diphenhydramine - For allergic reactions

- Antiseptic solution or ointment - To clean wounds or injuries

- Aloe Vera gel - to heal wounds or skin inflammation

Chapter 03 - Tips for Storage of Water and Food

In the face of adverse circumstances, it is important that you have enough food and water stored to keep you going for a long period of time. In this chapter I would share two more effective strategies with you,

Strategy# 9 - How to store water?

As water is more important to human life than food, let's discuss that first.

How much water do I need?

In ideas conditions, a single person consumes a gallon of water every day. Half a gallon is used for drinking purposes and the other half is used for hygiene.

How much water should you store for your survival?

According to experts, you should always have water you can consume for 3 days because after that you are likely to get help. But if some huge disaster strikes down, it's possible that you might not get aid for weeks and even month. So it is recommended that you store water that you can use in 2 weeks. This is just a start up. You can start by saving 2 weeks' worth water and then add up with time and money.

How can you store water for long periods of time?

If you are planning on storing water for long periods of time, you have to find a safe container to store the water in. You can use plastic bottles for storing water. Glass bottles are also good for storing water. You can store water in steel containers too but you would not be able to purify the water with Chlorine because the chemical will react with steel and cause rusting. Whatever container that you choose, make sure you can seal the container to prevent the water from harmful bacteria, germs and different dangerous pathogens that contaminate the water!

Water Barrels:

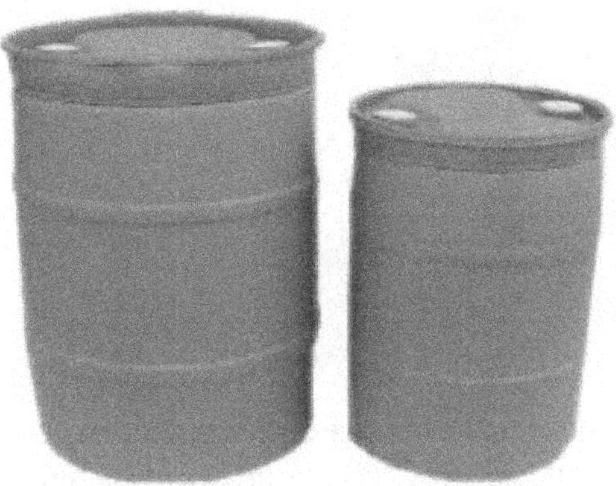

https://encrypted-tbn1.gstatic.com/images?q=tbn:ANd9GcSvI4-RRaBVhsZZL5Z0_7_gqozTzXOk5lDJO2C3sk7F088c1zI3

To store water for longer periods of time, you would need to get 55-gallon water barrels. They are made of food-grade plastic and you can seal them super tight too to keep the water from getting contaminated. These barrels are BPA-free and can keep the water or anything inside them safe from the UV radiations.

To keep these barrels, you would need a lot of space. These barrels are pretty expensive. One barrel can cost you up to $90. Also to fill them up, you would need a pump and a specialty drinking water hose. Also, these barrels and heavy and big and hence, not portable. One full barrel is 440 lbs.

Rain Barrels:

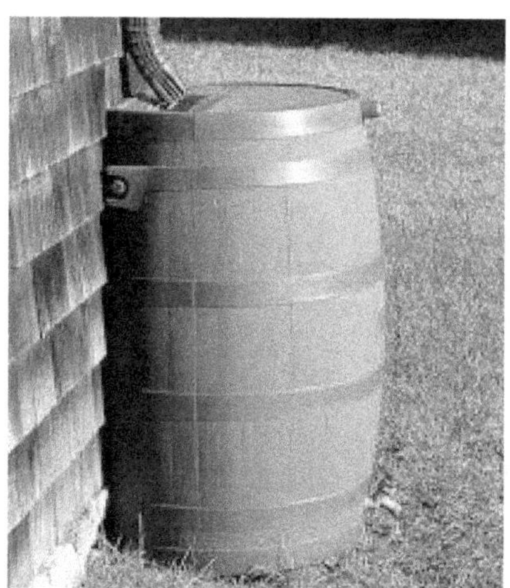

https://encrypted-tbn3.gstatic.com/images?q=tbn:ANd9GcQoZ_wXuOpgOe8GswxSrku-cirotOr_8h_sAp6qo-L1yEXT7AXB

To take advantage of the rain water, you can buy rain barrels too. They are eco-friendly and they don't cost a lot too. All you have to do is to put the rain barrel under the gutter pipe whenever it rains. The barrel would collect the rain water for you. You can store this water. But before you drink it, make sure you sanitize the water and purify it from all the germs and bacteria. You can use the rain water for hygiene and use the water in the water barrels for drinking purposes.

Also I have heard that there are some states that require you to get a permit before you start collecting rain water. And they would even charge you tax for that. Make sure you have checked all the information before you go ahead and start collecting rainwater. You don't want to do anything illegal, do you?

Now that you know how you can store water for prepping, the next effective strategy is about storing food.

Strategy# 10 - How to preserve and store food?

How can I store food?

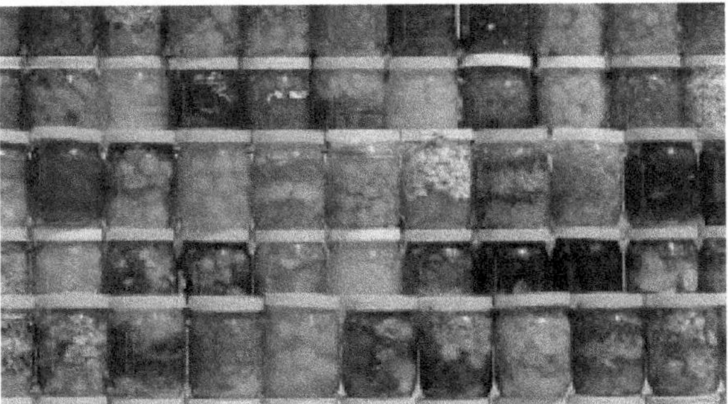

https://encrypted-tbn1.gstatic.com/images?q=tbn:ANd9GcR6sLQbZtyu2s7mGUiEvQZlrPEWn6G7KL28Vto1dm8Gn4p6n1HpUQ

There are many ways through which you can store and preserve food to prep for any disasters. You can store and preserve food for long periods of time by the following ways,

1. **Drying:**

   Drying is the easiest way if preserving food for long. This food preservation method doesn't require a lot of effort. Dry food items and store them for long period of time. As you know, mold grows in wet thing and moisture is vital for its growth so if you are using this method for the preservation of food, you can rest assured that your food is free from any bacteria and germs. Your dried food would stay for long without rotting or catching germs.

2. **Canning:**

   Canning is one of the traditional ways to preserve food. You can your food by cooking it partially so that all the bacteria and germs are dead. Then you can add certain additives like sugar syrup etc. After this you can clean the jars, dry them and put the partially cooked food items in the jars and seal them tight. You can keep these jars stored somewhere for a long time.

3. **Salt curing:**

   Salt curing is an old method by which you can preserve meat for a long time. Salt is used to keep the meat safe from bacteria because germs cannot survive in an environment where there is more than 10% of salt concentration. Meat is rubbed with a mixture of salt and sugar and then it is put in a jar or a pot that is shut super tight and kept where the temperature is cool

4. **Refrigeration:**

This is the most common way of preservation of food. You can keep cooked food and raw meat in the refrigerator to keep them safe for a long period of time. And when you need to eat the food, you can defrost it and cook it.

If you are able to keep enough food and water for your survival in the times of disasters, you would not have to worry about these basic human needs and you would be able to concentrate on other problems that you might face during harsh situations.

Chapter 04 - Train Your Mind for Survival Mentality

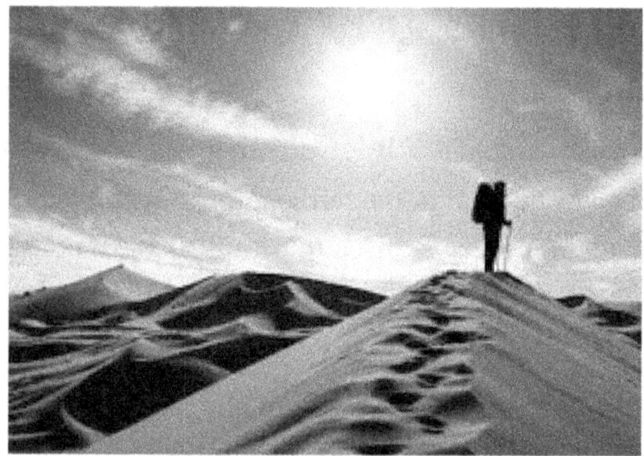

https://encrypted-tbno.gstatic.com/images?q=tbn:ANd9GcRpeKUNbW7P8hwW3oTEs-Iy3iISyIMeI_nyc9RK3XLMh6lhD4sf

The most important thing you need for survival is a calm and brave mind. If your mind is panicking and you cannot concentrate on surviving, you might not live long. In this chapter, I would give you 5 tips on how you can make a mind that will get you through all the adverse circumstances. But first there are a few things that I would like to discuss.

What is survival?

To be prepared to survive, to control your fears, to take control of your emotions, keep your ego in check. This is what survival is all about. It's not just about food, water and shelter. You have to have a sound mind and the ability to survive to actually survive a disaster.

Now, if you have knowledge about herbs, plants, how to make a fire, how to make a small hut etc, it would not be enough to keep you alive if you don't have the survival mentality. You have to be able to think clearly and make decisions fast to keep living in adverse circumstances.

If your mind is not strong enough, no amount of prepping would help you survive when a disaster strikes down.

How do you survive?

The answer to this is your mentality, how your mind confronts adverse situations. Survivors don't accept that they are helpless, they don't accept death even if they are so close to it. They have a **will to survive.** They refuse to let the circumstances decide if they would live or not. They choose to survive no matter what.

Without the **will to survive,** not even the most trained survivors would stand a chance against the circumstances. Knowing what you need to survive is very important but having a **will to survive** is the most important thing you need to survive.

A mindset that doesn't surrender and wants to live is the key to your survival in the most difficult circumstances.

Effects of fear on your mind:

There are two ways in which fear affects different people's mind,

1. Some people let the fear take over their mind. So much that they are unable to make any decisions on how to survive the situation. They are so scared that their ability to decide stops working. They close their eyes and give themselves to the fear and this kind of mindset leads them to their downfall.

2. There are people that use their fear to make quick decisions in order to rid themselves of the situation that is causing all the fear. These people allow their adrenaline to take over and this leads to hasty decisions. Because they don't get a chance to think clearly, they make wrong decisions and instead of solving the problem, create more problems for themselves.

Survival Mindset:

To survive in the most stressful circumstances, it is important that you control the flow of your thoughts, think calmly, don't panic and control your anxiety and your fears. Take control of your mind and be the master of yourself. If you let your mind control you, you would not survive. If you have a survival mindset and you can take a situation into your hands without panicking, you would be able to do things you never thought you could.

The last five tips on how to survive the most difficult of circumstances are probably the most important of all the tips that I have given you in this book. These tips include,

Strategy# 11 - Control your fear:

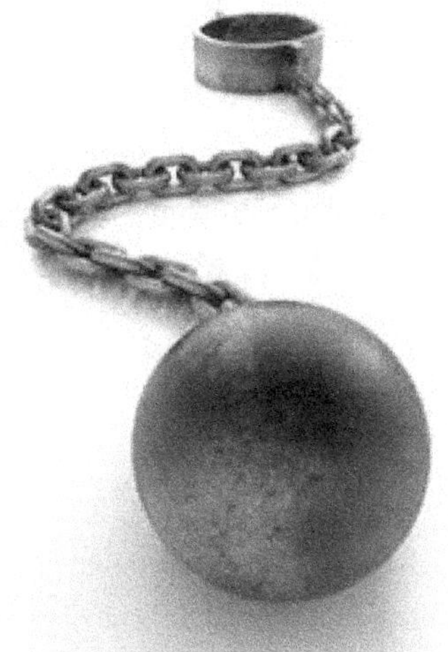

You have to control your fears and not panic. This is the first thing you should be able to do. When you face a life or death situation, you have to control your fear of ending up dead, because this very fear would get you killed. Just keep positive thoughts in your mind. Stop and breathe. Calm your mind. Clear your mind of all the negative thoughts and then start analyzing the situation and how you can handle it. You have to keep calm in the face of opposing circumstances, because panicking would only make things worse for you.

Strategy# 12 - Take control of your ego:

Don't panic and don't fear but don't overdo it. Drop that "nothing bad can happen to me" attitude of yours, because it can happen to you. Don't pretend that you have no fears and you can encounter anything without any hesitation or anxiety. That over-confidence can lead to your downfall. You have to be modest. Try to analyze your fears and train yourself in those areas until you are able to control them. Your ego can create bigger problems for you. So it is very important that you control your ego.

Strategy# 13 - Think of positive things:

To be able to think positively even in the face of extremely negative circumstances can lead to your victory. Develop a mindset that is all about positivity. Even if you are in a life or death situation, don't surrender to it. Just think positively and how you can survive the situation.

Strategy# 14 - Do not give in to your fears:

It is very important that you don't surrender to your fears, that you don't close your eyes when the situation is really, really difficult to cope with. The best way to survive any situation is to digest your fears, and try your best to fight the difficult situation. If you give in to your fears, you would end up dead.

Strategy# 15 - Keep training:

The last tip to survive any disaster is to be prepared all the time. Keep training yourself for the worst of circumstances. You can train yourself by practicing basic survival skills. Even if the circumstances are well and good, be prepared for the worst. The key to surviving sudden natural disasters is to be prepared all the time because who knows when a disaster strikes down.

Conclusion

To survive in the harshest of circumstances, one needs to be always prepared. You can do so by reading this book and understand everything. You can start practicing because disasters don't announce before they come. So if the circumstances become adverse suddenly, you have to be prepared for them beforehand.

You have to prep for different kinds of situations. In this book, you have learnt how you can tackle different survival situations. You have to store and preserve enough food to be able to survive times when you have no access to food. Human life cannot go on without water. You have to keep a considerable amount of water to keep you going until the circumstances are back to normal.

I hope that we never have to face circumstances that require these survival strategies and tips, but if we do, we would be prepared to face them. One thing that is really, really important is your mind set and your attitude in the face of adverse conditions. If you give in to the bad situations, it would be the death of you. If you want to live, you have to prepare a mind that is free from anxiety and that doesn't panic in the most panicky situations. **The Will to Survive** is the main key to surviving even the most difficult of situations. Good luck!

FREE Bonus Reminder

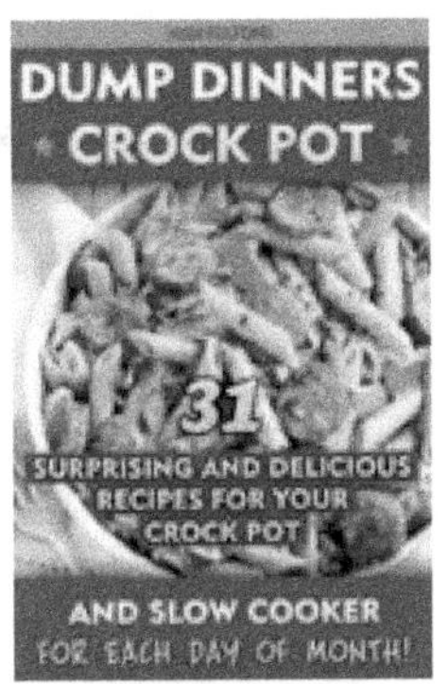

If you have not grabbed it yet, please go ahead and download your Free Ebook *"Dump Dinners Crock Pot: 31 Surprising And Delicious Recipes For Your Crock Pot And Slow Cooker For Each Day of Month!"*

Simply Click the Button Below

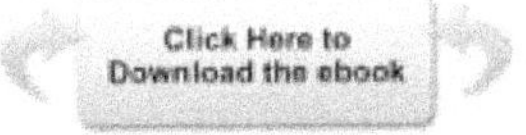

OR **Go to This Page**

http://easycookingideas.com/free

BONUS #2: More Free & Discounted Books

Do you want to receive more Free & Discounted Books?

We have a mailing list where we send out our new Books when they go free or with a discount on Kindle. Click on the link below to sign up for Free & Discount Book Promotions.

=> Sign Up for Free & Discount Book Promotions <=

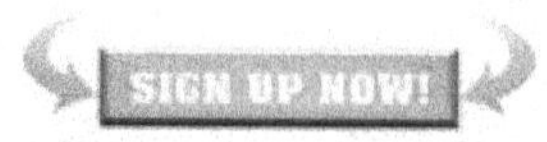

OR Go to this URL

http://zbit.ly/1WBb1Ek

www.ingramcontent.com/pod-product-compliance
Lightning Source LLC
Chambersburg PA
CBHW050805240726
48654CB00008B/636